Cambridge Elements ≡

Elements in Emergency Neurosurgery
edited by
Nihal Gurusinghe
Lancashire Teaching Hospital NHS Trust
Peter Hutchinson
University of Cambridge, Society of British Neurological Surgeons and Royal College of Surgeons of England
Ioannis Fouyas
Royal College of Surgeons of Edinburgh
Naomi Slator
North Bristol NHS Trust
Ian Kamaly-Asl
Royal Manchester Children's Hospital
Peter Whitfield
University Hospitals Plymouth NHS Trust

ADULT PATIENT WITH INTRAVENTRICULAR, PARAVENTRICULAR AND PINEAL REGION LESIONS

Mohamed Dablouk
Cork University Hospital and Royal College of Surgeons in Ireland

Mahmoud Kamel
Cork University Hospital

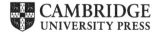

CAMBRIDGE
UNIVERSITY PRESS

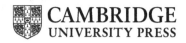

CAMBRIDGE
UNIVERSITY PRESS

Shaftesbury Road, Cambridge CB2 8EA, United Kingdom

One Liberty Plaza, 20th Floor, New York, NY 10006, USA

477 Williamstown Road, Port Melbourne, VIC 3207, Australia

314–321, 3rd Floor, Plot 3, Splendor Forum, Jasola District Centre,
New Delhi – 110025, India

103 Penang Road, #05–06/07, Visioncrest Commercial, Singapore 238467

Cambridge University Press is part of Cambridge University Press & Assessment,
a department of the University of Cambridge.

We share the University's mission to contribute to society through the pursuit of
education, learning and research at the highest international levels of excellence.

www.cambridge.org
Information on this title: www.cambridge.org/9781009487320

DOI: 10.1017/9781009487306

First published 2024

A catalogue record for this publication is available from the British Library.

ISBN 978-1-009-48732-0 Hardback
ISBN 978-1-009-48728-3 Paperback
ISSN 2755-0656 (online)
ISSN 2755-0648 (print)

Adult Patient with Intraventricular, Paraventricular and Pineal Region Lesions

Elements in Emergency Neurosurgery

DOI: 10.1017/9781009487306
First published online: December 2024

Mohamed Dablouk
Cork University Hospital and Royal College of Surgeons in Ireland

Mahmoud Kamel
Cork University Hospital

Author for correspondence: Mohamed Dablouk,
mohameddablouk@gmail.com

Abstract: Intraventricular lesions are uncommon, and they can arise from numerous structures around the ventricular system, including the ependyma, septum pellucidum and choroid plexus. Pineal region lesions may arise from the pineal gland parenchymal/supporting cells or glial cells of the midbrain/medial thalamus. Many of these lesions are either found incidentally or present with symptoms of hydrocephalus. Careful assessment of the clinical and radiological features of each case can help to narrow the differential diagnosis in this heterogenous group of tumours.

Keywords: brain tumour, neuro-oncology, neuro-endoscopy, pineal tumour, intraventricular tumour

ISBNs: 9781009487320 (HB), 9781009487283 (PB), 9781009487306 (OC)
ISSNs: 2755-0656 (online), 2755-0648 (print)

Contents

Key Points

- Intraventricular tumours are rare lesions.
- They can arise from numerous structures around the ventricular system, including the ependyma, septum pellucidum and choroid plexus.
- Many of these lesions are either asymptomatic and are found incidentally or present with symptoms of hydrocephalus.
- Careful assessment of the clinical and radiological features of each case can help to narrow the differential diagnosis.

1 Intraventricular Neoplasms

1.1 Differential Diagnosis of Intraventricular Lesions

The differential diagnosis for intraventricular lesions is broad. Table 1 provides some examples.

1.2 Case 1

A 38-year-old man presents to the emergency department with complaints of headache for the last two months. Examination reveals no neurological deficit. His MRI scan is shown in Figures 1 and 2.

Q1. What is the differential diagnosis?

- The differential diagnosis includes neoplastic lesions such as choroid plexus papilloma and meningioma, and vascular lesions such as arteriovenous malformation (AVM) or cavernoma.

Q2. What will you advise this patient?

- Given the diagnostic uncertainty, the patient is offered the options of radiological surveillance or surgical resection. He decides to undergo surgical resection.

Q3. What approaches can be used to target this lesion?

- Lesions of the lateral atrium can be approached through the interparietal sulcus approach, posterior temporal approach or the inferior temporal approach. The posterior transcallosal approach can provide better access to the medial atrium.

The patient undergoes a right temporal craniotomy and the lesion is resected via a posterior temporal approach. An external ventricular drain is left temporarily and removed after 48 hours (Figure 3). Post-operative MRI reveals complete excision (Figures 4 and 5). Pathological examination of the lesion reveals features consistent with a cavernous malformation.

Table 1 Intraventricular lesions (SEGA = subependymal
giant cell astrocytoma)

Origin	Tumour
Ventricular wall/septum pellucidum	Ependymoma
	Central neurocytoma
	SEGA
Choroid plexus lesion	Choroid plexus papilloma
	Choroid plexus carcinoma
Other	Meningioma
	Metastasis
	Colloid cyst
	Glioma

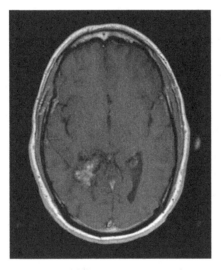

Figure 1 Axial T1 post-contrast image

Q4. What are the potential complications of this approach?

• During the posterior temporal approach, care must be taken not to injure the inferior anastomotic vein (of Labbe). If the mastoid air cells are entered, they must be waxed to prevent post-operative CSF leak. Care must be taken when planning the approach to prevent injury to the optic radiation, thus avoiding subsequent visual field defects.

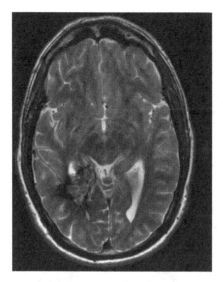

Figure 2 Axial T2 image

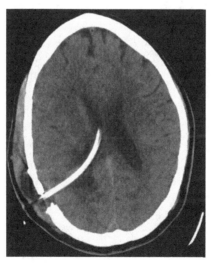

Figure 3 Post-operative CT image. An external ventricular drainage catheter is demonstrated within the right lateral ventricle

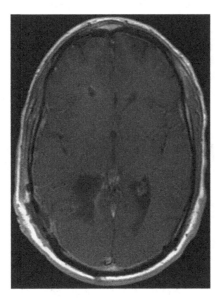

Figure 4 Post-operative T1 post-contrast image. No residual enhancement is demonstrated

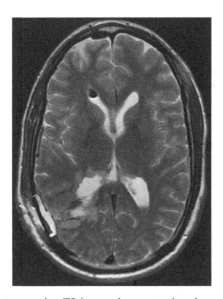

Figure 5 Post-operative T2 image demonstrating the operative tract. A small-volume pneumocephalus is seen

1.3 Case 2

An 18-year-old man with a previous diagnosis of migraine presents with a three day history of profuse vomiting and headache. He is admitted to his local hospital and a non-enhanced CT brain is performed (Figures 6 and 7).

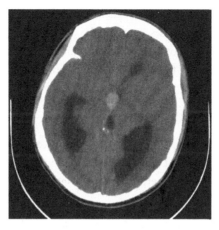

Figure 6 Axial non-enhanced CT at the level of the foramen of Monro

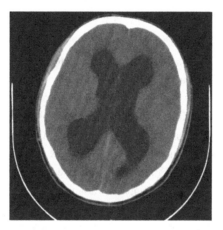

Figure 7 Axial non-enhanced CT

Q1. What are the important radiological features demonstrated in these images?

- This CT brain reveals a well-circumscribed hyperdense lesion in the anterior third ventricle, consistent with a colloid cyst. There is associated enlargement of the lateral ventricles, transependymal oedema and sulcal effacement, suggestive of acute obstructive hydrocephalus.

He is transferred to the neurosurgical unit. Upon arrival, he experiences a rapid decline in his level of consciousness.

Q2. What are your priorities in the management of this patient?

- This patient should be managed using the ABCD approach. The primary concern in an obtunded neurosurgical patient is the airway – anaesthetic support should be sought early in this case as the patient's neurological condition has acutely declined. Once the airway is secure and the patient's haemodynamic status is stable, urgent treatment of the cause of neurological decline (in this case, hydrocephalus secondary to the colloid cyst) is indicated.

Q3. What are the surgical options for the treatment of this pathology? When should surgery be performed?

- In general, the options are either CSF diversion or excision of the cyst. Given this patient's young age, it was felt that resection of the cyst would be the more appropriate option. Emergency surgery should be performed due to this patient's neurological status.

Q4. Describe the different approaches that can be used in this case.

- Excision of this colloid cyst can be performed via transcallosal, transcortical or endoscopic approaches. These approaches are described in further detail later in this element.

The patient is immediately taken to theatre, where he undergoes a craniotomy and transcortical transforaminal excision of the lesion, which is confirmed to be a colloid cyst. He makes an excellent neurological recovery. He develops a small pseudomeningocele at the wound, which resolves without intervention. He is discharged home in good condition. Follow-up CT brain reveals complete excision of the lesion, as seen in Figures 8 and 9 (note: although MRI is preferred for post-operative imaging in the majority of cases, colloid cysts can be more easily seen on CT and their MRI signal is variable).

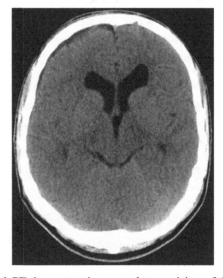

Figure 8 Axial CT demonstrating complete excision of the colloid cyst

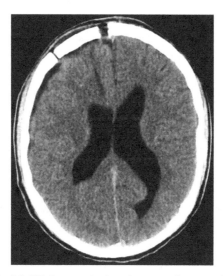

Figure 9 Axial CT demonstrating the operative tract in the right frontal lobe

Q4. What anatomical structures are potentially at risk during this surgery? What neurological deficits can occur as a result?

- Injury to the fornix is a feared complication of surgery for colloid cysts. Forniceal injury can result in significant short-term memory problems, which can be quite debilitating and can impede upon a patient's ability to lead an independent life.

1.4 Approaches to the Ventricular System

1.4.1 Endoscopic

The indications for endoscopic surgery have expanded over time. It is particularly well described for the removal of colloid cysts as the consistency and vascularity of these lesions lends itself well to endoscopic techniques. The role of endoscopy may be more limited for more solid/fibrous or more haemorrhagic lesions [1, 2]. Image guidance techniques can be integrated into the surgical workflow for endoscopic surgery; both electromagnetic and optical navigation systems can be used with most modern endoscope systems.

Colloid Cyst/Tumour Removal

- Pros
  - o Minimise brain trauma
  - o Less memory impairment

o Faster recovery, shorter hospital stay

o Narrow tract from ventricles to subdural space

- Cons

  o Difficult to achieve haemostasis

  o Poor bimanual surgery

  o Difficulty removing larger tumours

  o Equipment costs, learning costs

Tumour Biopsy

- Should be considered in situations where tumour resection may not be necessary or when diagnosis alters treatment approach (e.g. marker-negative germ cell tumours, infiltrative hypothalamic glioma, Langerhans cell histiocytosis).
- Simultaneous tumour biopsy and endoscopic third ventriculostomy (ETV) is feasible.

Post-Operative Considerations

- Ventricular drainage can be used for intracranial pressure monitoring or allowing egress of bloody CSF.
- Duration of drainage/monitoring is guided by individual clinical scenario.

1.4.2 Open

Approaches to the Lateral Ventricle

Anterior Transcallosal Approach

This approach is useful for lesions arising in the body of the lateral ventricle. Cortical veins draining into the sagittal sinus can be an obstacle and therefore pre-operative angiographic imaging can be of use. The details of the approach are as follows.

- Position: supine with slight flexion or lateral with affected hemisphere down.
- Incision: coronal incision anterior to coronal suture.
- Craniotomy: centred anterior to coronal suture; midline exposure up to sagittal sinus.
- Dura opened and reflected medially up to sinus.
- Once midline reached, follow falx to depth.
- Arachnoid below falx may be adherent – divide carefully to avoid injury to cingulate gyri.

- Once corpus callosum is reached, entry into ventricle takes place between pericallosal arteries.
- Callosotomy 2–3 cm just posterior to genu, slightly off midline and towards ventricle of interest.
- Orientation is confirmed by locating choroid plexus and thalamostriate vein.

Interparietal Sulcus Approach (Posterior Trans-Sulcal Approach)

This is a preferred route to the atrium of the lateral ventricle. Again, pre-operative angiographic imaging can help with identifying crossing veins. The patient is placed in the three-quarter prone position with the parietal region highest in the field. Once the craniotomy and durotomy are performed, dissection along the interparietal sulcus allows entry into the atrium.

Posterior Transcallosal Approach

This approach is useful for access to the roof and medial atrium of the lateral ventricles via splitting of the corpus callosum. It is not suitable for lesions of the lateral atrium or in patients with pre-operative homonymous hemianopia.

- Position: three-quarter prone position, parietal area of interest in dependent position.
- Craniotomy: from posterior edge of postcentral gyrus to 4 cm anterior, exposes sagittal sinus.
- Dissection along falx; pericallosal arteries and splenium identified.
- Splenium incised lateral to midline to enter the atrium.

Posterior Temporal Approach

This approach is useful for tumours located laterally in the atrium. Care must be taken not to injure the vein of Labbe. The optic radiation is also at risk of injury with this approach.

- Position: supine with head turned at least 60 degrees, or lateral.
- Craniotomy: exposes posterior temporal region just above plane with transverse sinus.
- Incision in posterior middle/inferior temporal gyrus and dissection to enter atrium.
- Inferior temporal bone and mastoid air cells can be removed to modify exposure on the dominant side – ensure watertight dural closure and waxing of air cells.

Inferior Temporal Approach

The inferior temporal approach is useful for accessing the temporal horn or the lateral atrium in the dominant hemisphere.

- Position: supine with head turned 45 degrees and slightly extended.
- Incision: reverse question mark.
- Craniotomy exposes the temporal lobe.
- Cortical incision in middle/inferior temporal gyrus or through inferior temporal sulcus to enter ventricle.

Approaches to the Anterior Third Ventricle

The transcallosal approach to the third ventricle is a continuation of the approach used to access the lateral ventricles. It can be used for lesions at or posterior to the foramen of Monro.

Transforaminal and Interforniceal Approaches

These approaches are useful to access the anterior third ventricle. They can be particularly useful in cases where the foramen of Monro has been dilated by the lesion. The choroidal fissure can be opened along the plane of the taenia fornicis to expand the foramen (Figure 10), although this approach may increase the risk of forniceal injury. The interforniceal approach is best used in patients who have a cavum septum pellucidum.

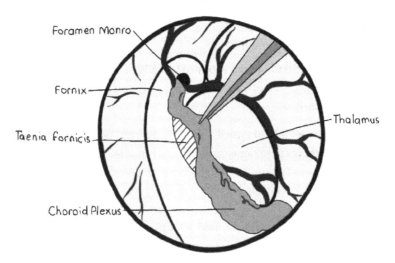

Figure 10 Transchoroidal approach to the third ventricle – the taenia fornicis is opened to expand the foramen of Monro

Lateral Subfrontal Approach

This is a useful approach for midline suprasellar and anterior third ventricular lesions.

- Position: supine.
- Incision: bicoronal/unilateral frontotemporal.
- Craniotomy: pterional craniotomy, low on orbital ridge.
- Subfrontal dissection is performed; once past planum sphenoidale the optic nerve/chiasm and internal carotid arteries (ICAs) are visualised.
- Lamina terminalis may need to be opened.

Approaches to the Posterior Third Ventricle

Transcallosal Transvelum Interpositum Approach

In this approach, the lateral ventricle is entered via the transcallosal approach. The choroid plexus is dissected medially through the taenia fornicis to separate it from the fornix. Once the choroid plexus is reflected laterally, the velum interpositum, internal cerebral vein (ICV) and medial posterior choroidal arteries are visualised. A plane can be developed between the ICVs to expose the third ventricle. The third ventricular choroid plexus is then separated in the midline to gain entry into the third ventricle.

Supracerebellar Infratentorial Approach

This approach is well suited for midline tumours in the pineal region. It is not optimal for tumours that infiltrate laterally or superiorly above the tentorium.

- Position: sitting/three-quarter prone/prone.
- Midline incision, wide suboccipital craniotomy exposing transverse sinus/ torcula.
- Dural opening based superiorly.
- Midline cerebellar bridging veins should be coagulated and divided; arachnoid is dissected.
- The precentral cerebellar vein connects vermis to vein to Galen – can be sacrificed.

Occipital Transtentorial Approach

This is a useful approach for pineal or posterior third ventricle lesions with supratentorial or infratentorial components. Bridging veins are seen infrequently along the medial occipital lobe.

- Position: sitting or semi-prone.
- Incision: trapdoor incision based inferiorly and crossing midline.
- Craniotomy: exposes midline and transverse sinus.
- Durotomy based on sinuses.
- Transection of tentorium from posterior to anterior; incise proximally and proceed in a line approximately 1 cm off midline towards tentorial edge.
- Falx can be cut approximately 1 cm anterior to insertion of vein of Galen, after coagulation/clip ligation of inferior sagittal sinus.
- Splenium can be gently retracted upwards to enhance exposure.

Complications of Lateral/Third Ventricular Surgery

Cognitive deficits may result from corpus callosum disconnection. These can be seen in up to 75% of cases and tend to resolve within three weeks, although permanent changes are seen in 5–10% of cases. The severity correlates with the length of the callosotomy. Symptoms can include disturbed consciousness, transient mutism, memory impairment, apathy, incontinence, disinhibition and contralateral leg weakness.

Seizures are more common in transcortical procedures [3]; however, retraction injuries can also cause post-operative seizures.

Hydrocephalus at presentation is common and can persist following resection in up to a third of patients.

2 Pineal Region Neoplasms

2.1 Case 3

An 18-year-old lady presents following an episode of collapse. She describes a history of headache and left-sided visual disturbance over the preceding two weeks. Examination reveals no focal neurological deficit. Her CT and MRI brain are shown in Figures 11 and 12.

Q1. Describe the pertinent findings on the images shown in Figures 11 and 12. What is the differential diagnosis?

- The post-contrast CT reveals a heterogenous lesion centred in the posterior third ventricle in the region of the pineal gland. The lesion is solid/cystic and there are some central areas of calcification. The MRI further demonstrates these findings, and also reveals that the lesion extends into the right ambient cistern and extends superiorly to the roof of the third ventricle. There is mild associated hydrocephalus.

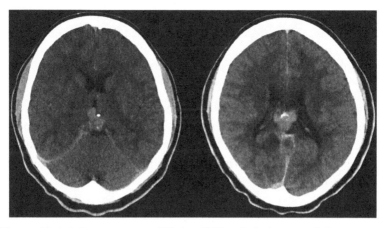

Figure 11 Axial post-contrast CT. A solid/cystic lesion containing areas of calcification is demonstrated in the posterior third ventricle

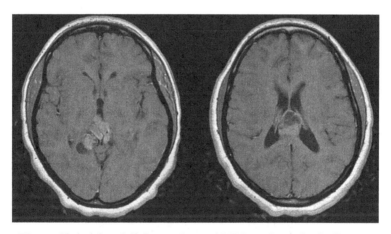

Figure 12 Axial gadolinium-enhanced MRI confirms the findings of a heterogenous posterior third ventricle tumour. The deep venous structures are closely related to the lesion

- The differential diagnosis includes a pineal tumour (germ cell tumour, pineal cell tumour, glial cell tumour), tectal plate tumour or inferior thalamic tumour.

Q2. What further investigations are necessary?

- An MRI of the rest of the neuro-axis is obtained, which reveals no other lesions. Tests for serum tumour markers and CSF are sent – tumour markers are negative, and CSF cytology reveals evidence of malignant cells.

The patient is discussed at the neuro-oncology multidisciplinary team (MDT) meeting and given these findings it is recommended that a tissue diagnosis is obtained.

Q3. What are the surgical options in this case?

- Biopsy versus surgical resection. Biopsy can be performed either endo-scopically or stereotactically. There are several microsurgical approaches to the pineal region/posterior third ventricle, the most well established being the supracerebellar infratentorial (SCIT) approach and the occipital transtentorial approach.

The patient initially undergoes stereotactic biopsy via a right parietal burrhole. Histopathological examination is consistent with CNS WHO grade 4 pine-oblastoma. Following further MDT meeting discussion, she undergoes debulk-ing of the lesion via a right-sided occipital transtentorial approach. She undergoes adjuvant treatment with medical and radation oncology. Her post-operative imaging at three months is shown in Figure 13.

2.2 Clinical Points

The pineal region can host a diverse group of tumours. They may arise from pineal parenchymal cells, supporting cells of the pineal gland or glial cells of the midbrain/medial thalamus. Numerous surgical approaches to the pineal region have been described, from Dandy's interhemispheric approach and Van

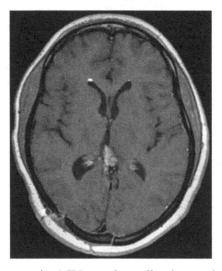

Figure 13 Post-operative MRI reveals small-volume enhancing residual

Table 2 Symptoms of pineal region masses

Site of compression	Symptom
Brainstem	Parinaud syndrome
Superior cerebellar peduncle	Ataxia, dysmetria
Inferior colliculus	Hearing disturbance

Wagenen's transventricular approach to the more often used supracerebellar infratentorial and occipital transtentorial approaches [4].

Generally, these tumours can be grouped into four main categories:

- Germ cell tumours
- Pineal cell tumours
- Glial cell tumours
- Miscellaneous (wide range of histology)

Patients with pineal region tumours can present with symptoms due to hydrocephalus, compression (Table 2) or, less frequently, endocrine dysfunction.

The initial investigation of patients with pineal region tumours is of crucial importance as not all these patients will require intervention in the form of surgery (Figure 14) [5]. Alpha fetoprotein (AFP) and beta-human chorionic gonadotropin (b-HCG) are markers of germ cell malignancy that can be measured in serum and CSF. Elevation of these markers is pathognomonic for the presence of malignant germ cell elements.

In patients with marker-positive tumours, measurement of these levels can also be helpful to monitor treatment response and to assess for recurrence.

2.3 Pre-operative Considerations

2.3.1 Surgical Anatomy

Most of these tumours arise from or attach to the undersurface of the velum interpositum and tela choroidea. They are related to the choroid plexus, deep venous system and posterior choroidal arteries. Typically, the venous structures surround the periphery of the tumour. Key aspects of the anatomy which should be considered are the relationship to the third ventricle and quadrigeminal cistern, and the lateral and superior extent of the tumour.

2.3.2 Hydrocephalus

Pre-operative CSF diversion treats symptomatic hydrocephalus and allows CSF sampling for tumour markers. Some mildly symptomatic patients may not

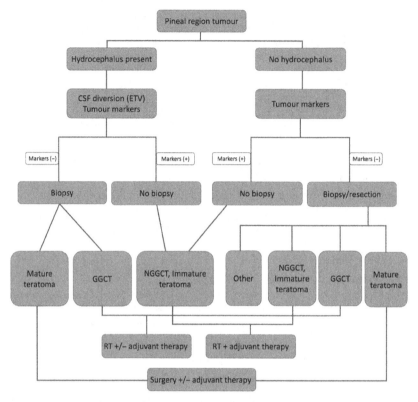

Figure 14 Workup of pineal region tumours. Adapted from: Zaazoue MA, Goumnerova LC. Pineal region tumors: a simplified management scheme. Childs Nerv Syst. 2016;32(11):2041–5

require CSF diversion as complete tumour removal can result in resolution of the hydrocephalus.

Endoscopic third ventriculostomy (ETV) can result in a gradual reduction in intracranial pressure and symptom resolution without the potential complications of ventriculoperitoneal shunt insertion; however, it is contraindicated in some cases (e.g. the tumour occupies the floor of the third ventricle; unfavourable relationship between the third ventricle floor and basilar artery).

2.3.3 Biopsy versus Resection

Histology is critical for guiding treatment decisions. The options for obtaining tissue are biopsy (endoscopic/stereotactic) or open surgery. The various pros and cons are detailed in Table 3. It is important to note that mixed tumours of the pineal region may occur, and therefore smaller tissue samples

Table 3 Advantages and disadvantages of different methods of biopsy

	Open surgery	**Stereotactic biopsy**	**Endoscopic biopsy**
Pros	More extensive sampling Allows for tumour removal	Ease of performance	Allows for simultaneous ETV
Cons	Higher morbidity	Risk of haemorrhage Limited tissue	Difficult haemostasis Limited tissue

may sometimes lead to sampling error by only evaluating one component of a mixed tumour.

2.4 Outcomes

Benign tumours of the pineal region/posterior third ventricle (e.g. meningioma, teratoma, pilocytic astrocytoma) are best treated with surgical resection. These tumours may be encapsulated, which can aid in minimising surgical morbidity.

Germinoma is the most common tumour in the pineal region. Most occur in males in the second or third decade of life. These tumours are radiosensitive – long-term survival rates of 80–90% are achievable with radiotherapy to the tumour and ventricular system [6]. Whole-brain radiotherapy is reserved for non-responders to first-line radiotherapy and chemotherapy.

Non-germinomatous germ cell tumours carry a poor prognosis. Most occur in young patients, with two-thirds being diagnosed between 10 and 21 years of age [7]. Tumours included in this category are endodermal sinus tumour, choriocarcinoma and embryonal carcinoma. Most can be diagnosed based on tumour markers, and biopsy is often unnecessary. Combination treatment with chemotherapy and radiotherapy affords the best outcomes.

Pineal parenchymal tumours exist along a spectrum, ranging from benign pineocytoma to aggressive pineoblastoma. Pineocytomas, although seen in all age groups, are more common in adults between 30 and 60 years. Pineoblastoma is more common in children [8]. The characteristics of these tumours are outlined in Table 4.

Pineal astrocytoma is poorly characterised within the existing literature [9]. These tumours are often cystic. Gross total resection is achievable and often results in a cure. Rarely, glioblastoma may occur in the pineal region.

Table 4 Pineal parenchymal tumours

Tumour	Features/treatment
Pineocytoma	Benign; radical surgery +/− radiation for residual
PPTID (pineal parenchymal tumour of intermediate differentiation)	Behaviour can be unpredictable; radical resection favoured
Pineoblastoma	Aggressive, prone to metastasis; radical surgery with radiation +/− chemotherapy

2.5 Approaches to the Pineal Region

2.5.1 Supracerebellar Infratentorial Approach (SCIT)

There are several benefits to this approach:

- Approaches the centre of the tumour (which begins at midline and grows eccentrically).
- Approaches inferior to the velum interpositum and deep venous system (tumour is often adherent to these structures).
- No normal tissue is violated along the operative corridor.

2.5.2 Occipital Transtentorial/Interhemispheric Transcallosal Approach

These approaches can be helpful in the following circumstances:

- Tumour extends superiorly, involves/destroys posterior corpus callosum or deflects deep venous system dorsolaterally.
- Tumour extends laterally towards the trigone.
- Tumour extends inferiorly into the quadrigeminal plate.
- Tumour displaces venous system ventrally (occurs infrequently).

References

1. Rocque BG. Neuroendoscopy for intraventricular tumor resection. World Neurosurg. 2016;90:619–20.
2. Kim MH. Transcortical endoscopic surgery for intraventricular lesions. J Korean Neurosurg Soc. 2017;60(3):327–34.
3. Eichberg DG, Sedighim S, Buttrick S, Komotar RJ. Postoperative seizure rate after transcortical resection of subcortical brain tumors and colloid cysts: a single surgeon's experience. Cureus. 2018;10(1):e2115.
4. Behari S, Garg P, Jaiswal S, Nair A, Naval R, Jaiswal AK. Major surgical approaches to the posterior third ventricular region: a pictorial review. J Pediatr Neurosci. 2010;5(2):97–101.
5. Zaazoue MA, Goumnerova LC. Pineal region tumors: a simplified management scheme. Childs Nerv Syst. 2016;32(11):2041–5.
6. Villano JL, Propp JM, Porter KR et al. Malignant pineal germ-cell tumors: an analysis of cases from three tumor registries. Neuro Oncol. 2008;10(2):121–30.
7. Jennings MT, Gelman R, Hochberg F. Intracranial germ-cell tumors: natural history and pathogenesis. J Neurosurg. 1985;63(2):155–67.
8. Favero G, Bonomini F, Rezzani R. Pineal gland tumors: a review. Cancers (Basel). 2021;13(7):13.
9. Choque-Velasquez J, Resendiz-Nieves J, Jahromi BR et al. Long-term survival outcomes of pineal region gliomas. J Neurooncol. 2020;148(3):651–8.

Cambridge Elements ☰

Emergency Neurosurgery

Nihal Gurusinghe
Lancashire Teaching Hospital NHS Trust

Professor Nihal Gurusinghe is a Consultant Neurosurgeon at the Lancashire Teaching Hospitals NHS Trust. He is on the Executive Council of the Society of British Neurological Surgeons as the Lead for NICE (National Institute for Health and Care Excellence) guidelines relating to neurosurgical practice. He is also an examiner for the UK and International FRCS examinations in Neurosurgery.

Peter Hutchinson
University of Cambridge, Society of British Neurological Surgeons and Royal College of Surgeons of England

Peter Hutchinson BSc MBBS FFSEM FRCS(SN) PhD FMedSci is Professor of Neurosurgery and Head of the Division of Academic Neurosurgery at the University of Cambridge, and Honorary Consultant Neurosurgeon at Addenbrooke's Hospital. He is Director of Clinical Research at the Royal College of Surgeons of England and Meetings Secretary of the Society of British Neurological Surgeons.

Ioannis Fouyas
Royal College of Surgeons of Edinburgh

Ioannis Fouyas is a Consultant Neurosurgeon in Edinburgh. His clinical interests focus on the treatment of complex cerebrovascular and skull base pathologies. His academic endeavours concentrate in the field of cerebrovascular pathophysiology. His passion is technical surgical training, fulfilled in collaboration with the Royal College of Surgeons of Edinburgh. Finally, he pursues Undergraduate Neuroscience teaching, with a particular focus on functional Neuroanatomy.

Naomi Slator
North Bristol NHS Trust

Naomi Slator FRCS (SN) is a Consultant Spinal Neurosurgeon based at North Bristol NHS Trust. She has a specialist interest in Complex Spine alongside Cranial and Spinal Trauma. She completed her neurosurgical training in Birmingham and a six-month Fellowship in CSF and Trauma (2019). She then went on to complete her Spinal Fellowship in Leeds (2020) before moving to the southwest to take up her consultant post.

Ian Kamaly-Asl
Royal Manchester Children's Hospital

Ian Kamaly-Asl is a full time paediatric neurosurgeon and Honorary Chair at Royal Manchester Children's Hospital. He trained in North Western Deanery with fellowships at Boston Children's Hospital and Sick Kids in Toronto. Ian is a member of council of The Royal College of Surgeons of England and The SBNS where he is lead for mentoring and tackling oppressive behaviours.

Peter Whitfield
University Hospitals Plymouth NHS Trust

Professor Peter Whitfield is a Consultant Neurosurgeon at the South West Neurosurgical Centre, University Hospitals Plymouth NHS Trust. His clinical interests include vascular neurosurgery, neuro oncology and trauma. He has held many roles in postgraduate neurosurgical education and is President of the Society of British Neurological Surgeons. Peter has published widely, and is passionate about education, training and the promotion of clinical research.

About the Series

Elements in Emergency Neurosurgery is intended for trainees and practitioners in Neurosurgery and Emergency Medicine as well as allied specialties all over the world. Authored by international experts, this series provides core knowledge, common clinical pathways and recommendations on the management of acute conditions of the brain and spine.

Cambridge Elements ≡

Emergency Neurosurgery

Elements in the Series

The Challenges of On-Call Neurosurgery
Abteen Mostofi, Marco Lee and Nihal Gurusinghe

Mild Traumatic Brain Injury including Concussion
Thomas D. Parker and Colette Griffin

Models for Delivering High Quality Emergency Neurosurgery in High Income Countries
Matthew A. Boissaud-Cooke, Marike Broekman, Jeroen van Dijck, Marco Lee and Paul Grundy

Acute Spontaneous Posterior Fossa Haemorrhage
Lauren Harris and Patrick Grover

Clinical Priority for Common Emergency and Urgent Conditions in Neurosurgery
Taha Lilo and Ioannis Fouyas

Management of Seizures in Neurosurgical Practice
Julie Woodfield and Susan Duncan

Cranial and Spinal Tuberculosis Infections including Acute Presentations
Veekshith Shetty and Pragnesh Bhatt

Spinal Discitis and Epidural Abscess
Damjan Veljanoski and Pragnesh Bhatt

Adult Patient with Intraventricular, Paraventricular and Pineal Region Lesions
Mohamed Dablouk and Mahmoud Kamel

A full series listing is available at: www.cambridge.org/EEMN

Printed in the United States
by Baker & Taylor Publisher Services